Antiparasitic Armaments

Pharmaceutical Innovations and Treatment Modalities

Cordelia Ashworth

Table of Contents

1 Introduction to Parasitology

Parasitology, the study of parasites, encompasses a vast and intricate world of organisms that rely on a host for survival. These organisms, ranging from microscopic protozoa to sizable helminths, exhibit remarkable diversity in their life cycles, habitats, and pathogenic mechanisms. Understanding this diversity is crucial for effective diagnosis and treatment. Their impact on global health is undeniable, affecting millions worldwide and contributing significantly to morbidity and mortality, particularly in developing nations.

The classification of parasites reflects this diversity. Protozoa, single-celled eukaryotes, are often categorized based on their motility and morphology, including flagellates, amoebas, ciliates, and sporozoa. Helminths, multicellular worms, are grouped into three major phyla: Platyhelminthes (flatworms, including flukes and tapeworms), Nematoda (roundworms), and Acanthocephala (thorny-headed worms). Each group presents unique challenges in terms of diagnosis, treatment, and control. The complex life cycles of many parasites, often involving multiple hosts and environmental stages, further complicate efforts to mitigate their impact.

Consider the global burden of parasitic diseases. Malaria, caused by Plasmodium species, remains a leading cause of mortality, particularly among children in sub-Saharan Africa. Soil-transmitted helminths, including hookworms, whipworms, and roundworms, affect billions worldwide, impacting physical and cognitive development, especially in children. Schistosomiasis, a debilitating disease caused by blood flukes, affects hundreds of millions in tropical and subtropical regions. These are just a few examples of the immense public health challenge posed by parasitic infections. The economic implications are substantial, affecting productivity, healthcare systems, and overall development.

Effective control strategies require a multifaceted approach, combining drug treatment with preventive measures. Improved sanitation, access to clean water, and vector control are essential in reducing transmission. Education plays a vital role in promoting hygiene practices and increasing community awareness. However, drug resistance is an emerging threat, requiring constant vigilance and the development of new therapeutic strategies. The complexity of parasite biology and the challenges of drug development highlight the need for a concerted global effort. This is especially important given the potential of emerging and neglected parasitic diseases. The continued evolution of parasites, their ability to develop resistance to current drugs and their exploitation of ecological niches makes them a constant threat to human health.

The development of new antiparasitic drugs is crucial in combating this global health threat. This requires a deep understanding of parasite biology, drug metabolism and drug interactions. Research continues to focus on identifying novel drug targets, improving drug delivery systems, and developing combination therapies to overcome resistance. These strategies will ultimately allow for more effective treatment and improved health outcomes. This chapter has only provided a brief overview, but it has laid the groundwork for a more thorough exploration of these vital topics in the chapters that follow. The battle against parasitic diseases is an ongoing and crucial endeavor. Understanding the scope of the problem, as this chapter outlines, is the first step in fighting back. The fight against parasites is a long-term and complex one, requiring sustained effort from researchers, healthcare professionals, and communities around the world.

1.1 Parasite Classification

Protozoa, the single-celled eukaryotes, represent a diverse group within the parasitic world. Among them, the apicomplexans, characterized by their apical complex – an organelle crucial for host cell invasion – are infamous for causing diseases like malaria (Plasmodium spp.)

and toxoplasmosis (Toxoplasma gondii). Their complex life cycles, often involving multiple hosts, pose significant challenges for treatment. Understanding their unique metabolic pathways and the intricacies of their interactions with host cells is essential for developing effective therapies. This necessitates targeted drug design, focusing on parasite-specific enzymes or pathways absent in the human host, minimizing adverse effects. Moreover, research continues to explore ways to interrupt their complex life cycles, targeting specific stages for maximal impact.

Next, we have the flagellates, a group including the notorious Trypanosoma brucei, the causative agent of African sleeping sickness. Their ability to evade the host's immune system through antigenic variation and their unique biochemical pathways make them particularly challenging therapeutic targets. Current treatment options for African trypanosomiasis often involve toxic drugs with significant side effects, underscoring the urgent need for safer and more effective alternatives. The development of new drugs requires a comprehensive understanding of the parasite's unique biology and the intricacies of its interactions with the host immune system. This might involve, for instance, developing drugs that target specific surface proteins involved in immune evasion. Furthermore, novel drug delivery systems might improve treatment efficacy by enhancing drug penetration and reducing systemic toxicity.

Helminths, or parasitic worms, constitute another major group, encompassing nematodes (roundworms), cestodes (tapeworms), and trematodes (flukes). Nematodes, such as Ascaris lumbricoides, Trichuris trichiura, and hookworms, cause significant morbidity and mortality, primarily affecting populations in developing countries. These infections can lead to malnutrition and anemia, significantly impacting economic productivity. The control measures include improved sanitation, hygiene practices, and effective anthelmintic drugs. However, drug resistance is a growing concern, necessitating innovative approaches, like the development of new drug classes with different mechanisms of action, or the exploration of combination therapies to overcome resistance.

Cestodes, like Taenia saginata (beef tapeworm) and Taenia solium (pork tapeworm), inhabit the human intestine, causing digestive issues and potential complications. Treatment usually involves praziquantel, a drug known for its broad-spectrum anthelminthic activity. However, its effectiveness can be impacted by factors such as the parasite's lifecycle stage and the host's immune response. Therefore, optimizing treatment strategies requires considering parasite species, patient characteristics, and the geographic context. The treatment for these parasites may involve surgery to remove the adult worms in specific cases. In addition, improved sanitation and hygiene measures are crucial to prevent infection.

Trematodes, a diverse group of flukes, cause a wide range of diseases depending on the species. Schistosoma spp., responsible for schistosomiasis, have a complex life cycle involving both intermediate and definitive hosts. Effective control requires targeting multiple points in the life cycle, often involving broad-based public health interventions. The treatment primarily employs praziquantel, but alternative therapies are actively researched due to the emergence of drug resistance and the need to address the associated morbidity. The development of new drugs or improvement in the existing ones with minimal side effects is the need of the hour. The efficacy of these drugs is highly impacted by the host's immune response.

Finally, ectoparasites, such as lice, ticks, and fleas, although not technically classified as internal parasites, are significant disease vectors. They can cause direct harm through infestations and transmit several pathogenic organisms. Effective control measures necessitate topical treatments, environmental management, and sometimes systemic medications depending on the severity and type of infestation. Integrated pest management strategies are important, especially for tackling vectors of more serious diseases. Resistance to insecticides is a major concern, necessitating a multi-pronged approach combining chemical and non-chemical control methods. Understanding the parasite's life cycle, host-parasite interactions and the development of targeted interventions are vital to the continued progress of effective antiparasitic treatments.

1.2 Global Parasite Burden

The sheer scale of parasitic infections globally is staggering. Millions suffer, countless more are at risk, and the economic impact reverberates across healthcare systems and national economies worldwide. Understanding this global parasite burden requires a multifaceted approach, going beyond simple infection rates. We must consider the complex interplay of factors driving this burden, ranging from socioeconomic disparities and environmental conditions to the limitations of current diagnostic tools and the ever-evolving nature of parasites themselves. This necessitates a nuanced perspective, one that acknowledges the disproportionate impact on vulnerable populations and the urgent need for innovative solutions.

Consider malaria, a disease that continues to claim hundreds of thousands of lives annually, primarily affecting children under five in sub-Saharan Africa. This devastation is not solely due to the parasite itself; it's worsened by poverty, inadequate sanitation, and limited access to effective treatment and prevention strategies. The consequences extend beyond immediate mortality; malaria's debilitating effects significantly hamper economic productivity, impacting educational attainment and perpetuating cycles of poverty across generations. Similarly, neglected tropical diseases, often grouped together due to their prevalence in low-income countries, present another significant piece of this global puzzle. These diseases, including schistosomiasis, soil-transmitted helminthiases, and lymphatic filariasis, cause widespread morbidity and impaired development, creating a heavy burden on healthcare resources and economic productivity within the affected regions.

The geographical distribution of these parasites is far from uniform. Tropical and subtropical regions bear the brunt of the burden, but parasitic infections are not confined to these areas. Climate change, facilitating the spread of vector-borne diseases, poses an escalating threat. Globalization and increased human migration further complicate the issue, enabling the movement of parasites across geographical boundaries and increasing the potential for outbreaks in previously unaffected regions. The consequences are significant; expanding the reach of infections often taxes already strained healthcare systems and overwhelms local resources, exacerbating the existing global health inequalities.

Furthermore, accurate assessment of the global parasite burden is a challenge itself. Many parasitic infections are asymptomatic or present with non-specific symptoms, making diagnosis difficult, particularly in resource-limited settings. Limited diagnostic capabilities, combined with poor surveillance systems, lead to underreporting and an inaccurate picture of the true extent of the problem. This underestimation hinders effective resource allocation and impedes the implementation of targeted interventions.

The economic costs associated with parasitic infections are substantial, encompassing direct healthcare costs, lost productivity due to illness and disability, and the cost of prevention and control programs. The indirect costs, including the impact on education, agricultural output, and overall economic development, are often even harder to quantify, yet equally significant. These economic burdens disproportionately impact developing nations, further widening the gap between wealthier and poorer countries. This necessitates a deeper understanding of the economic consequences, allowing for more strategic investments in research, development, and implementation of effective interventions.

Addressing this multifaceted problem requires a collaborative global effort. International collaborations, increased funding for research and development, improved diagnostic tools and surveillance systems, and strong health infrastructure are crucial. Educational campaigns to promote hygiene, sanitation and other preventative measures are equally important, as are the development and distribution of effective treatments and preventative measures, especially those targeting vulnerable populations. Only through a combined effort and commitment to tackling this global health challenge can we begin to reduce the immense suffering and economic burden caused by parasitic infections.

The path forward involves not only advancements in pharmaceuticals, but also substantial improvements in public health infrastructure and proactive community involvement. The fight against parasites is, ultimately, a fight for global health equity and economic progress.

2 Antiparasitic Drug Mechanisms

Many antiparasitic drugs target crucial metabolic pathways within the parasite, effectively disrupting their energy production and survival. For instance, metronidazole, used against anaerobic protozoa like Giardia lamblia, interferes with DNA synthesis by disrupting the parasite's electron transport chain, leading to cell death. This selective toxicity arises from the parasite's reliance on anaerobic metabolism, unlike the host's aerobic processes. Understanding these metabolic differences is fundamental to developing drugs that minimize harm to the host while maximizing efficacy against the parasite. The precise mechanisms of action of these drugs are continually being refined, particularly as we learn about the specific enzymes and pathways involved. This ongoing research is vital for overcoming drug resistance and developing new, more effective treatments.

Some drugs directly interfere with parasite reproduction, preventing them from multiplying and causing infection. These drugs frequently target crucial stages in the parasite's life cycle. For example, praziquantel, used against several types of flatworms (trematodes and cestodes), alters the parasite's cell membrane permeability, causing calcium influx and subsequent paralysis and death. The disruption of essential reproductive processes effectively limits the parasite population, aiding the host's immune system in clearing the remaining organisms. Moreover, the precise stage of the parasite life cycle that's targeted dictates the timing and frequency of drug administration. The effectiveness of such drugs hinges on a thorough understanding of the parasite's reproductive biology and its susceptibility to these targeted interventions.

Numerous antiparasitic drugs function by inhibiting the activity of specific enzymes essential for parasite survival. These enzymes may be involved in various processes such as protein synthesis, nucleic acid synthesis, or nutrient metabolism. For instance, ivermectin, a broad-spectrum antiparasitic drug, primarily targets glutamate-gated chloride channels found in invertebrate parasites, causing paralysis and death. This precise targeting of specific parasite enzymes minimizes the effects on the host. The development of drugs which target such unique enzymes is paramount in designing therapies that are both highly effective and have minimal side effects on the human host. Furthermore, understanding the three-dimensional structure of these enzymes is crucial in designing drugs that fit perfectly into the active site, thus blocking their activity.

The complexity of parasitic infections necessitates a multi-faceted approach to treatment. Success often relies not on a single drug but on a carefully considered combination of approaches. In many cases, combination therapies are employed to overcome drug resistance and reduce the risk of adverse effects. For example, the treatment of malaria often involves artemisinin-based combination therapies (ACTs), combining artemisinin derivatives with other anti-malarial drugs. This strategy helps prevent the emergence of resistant parasite strains and increases the overall effectiveness of treatment. Combining different classes of antiparasitic drugs that target different metabolic pathways or life cycle stages is usually more effective. The rationale behind combination therapies is to synergistically impact the parasite, making it harder to develop resistance. This carefully balanced approach, while seemingly more complex, significantly improves the efficacy of treatment and patient outcomes.

The development of new antiparasitic drugs is crucial in combating the increasing problem of drug resistance. Research focuses on identifying novel drug targets within the parasite, exploiting their unique biochemical pathways and characteristics to develop specific inhibitors. This involves identifying vulnerabilities in parasite biology, employing techniques such as genomics and proteomics to discover new drug targets. The use of advanced technologies such as high-throughput screening and computer-aided drug design also allows for efficient identification of potential drug candidates. Careful assessment of the drug's pharmacokinetic and pharmacodynamic properties is paramount in ensuring both efficacy and safety. Furthermore, preclinical testing, both in vitro and in vivo, is essential for evaluating the effectiveness and toxicity of a new antiparasitic agent before it can proceed to clinical trials in humans. Such rigorous testing is a crucial step in bringing new, effective antiparasitic treatments to those in need.

2.1 Targeting Metabolic Pathways

Targeting metabolic pathways offers a potent strategy in antiparasitic drug design. Many parasites rely on metabolic processes fundamentally different from their human hosts, creating exploitable vulnerabilities. For instance, the unique folate biosynthesis pathway in certain protozoa, like Plasmodium falciparum, the causative agent of malaria, is a well-established drug target. Sulfonamides and dihydrofolate reductase inhibitors, by blocking key steps in this pathway, effectively hinder parasite growth and replication, demonstrating the success of this approach.

Exploiting differences in energy metabolism represents another avenue. Many parasites, especially anaerobic helminths, depend on glycolysis or other anaerobic pathways for energy production, unlike humans who primarily use aerobic respiration. Drugs targeting these anaerobic pathways, while sparing human cells, could prove highly effective. This strategy requires careful consideration to minimize off-target effects and potential toxicity. We must thoroughly understand the parasite's metabolic network to identify specific points of intervention with minimal impact on the host.

Beyond glycolysis, other metabolic pathways offer fertile ground for drug discovery. For example, the synthesis of fatty acids or sterols, essential components of parasite membranes, are often distinct from human pathways. Interfering with these pathways could disrupt membrane integrity and lead to parasite death. This approach has shown promise in treating certain parasitic infections, particularly those caused by trypanosomes and leishmania. Research continues to unveil novel targets and refine the selectivity of drugs targeting these pathways.

However, the effectiveness of this strategy hinges on accurate identification and validation of potential targets. Advanced techniques such as genomics, metabolomics, and proteomics play crucial roles in mapping parasite metabolic networks and pinpointing enzymes or pathways uniquely essential for parasite survival. This detailed understanding allows researchers to design drugs specifically targeting these pathways, maximizing efficacy while minimizing side effects. Computational modeling and in silico drug design are also increasingly valuable tools in this process, helping to predict the efficacy and selectivity of potential drug candidates before costly and time-consuming in vivo testing.

Furthermore, the development of drugs targeting metabolic pathways often requires overcoming challenges related to drug delivery. Many parasites reside within host cells or tissues, creating barriers to drug penetration. Enhancing drug bioavailability and penetration is critical for effective treatment. This necessitates designing drugs with improved pharmacokinetic and pharmacodynamic properties, including better absorption, distribution, metabolism, and excretion. Formulating drugs in suitable delivery systems, such as nanoparticles or liposomes, could also improve drug efficacy.

The emergence of drug resistance poses a significant threat to the long-term effectiveness of antiparasitic drugs targeting metabolic pathways. Parasites can develop resistance through mutations in the drug target or changes in drug transport mechanisms. This necessitates a multifaceted strategy involving drug combinations, careful monitoring of resistance patterns, and the development of new drugs with novel mechanisms of action. Proactive surveillance and the development of rapid diagnostic tools are essential to detect and manage the spread of drug-resistant parasites.

In conclusion, targeting metabolic pathways remains a significant area of focus in antiparasitic drug development. The inherent differences between parasite and human metabolism offer unique opportunities for selective drug action. However, a comprehensive understanding of the parasite's metabolic network is essential to ensure the success of this strategy. Challenges associated with drug delivery and the emergence of drug resistance need to be actively addressed through innovative research and careful monitoring. Further research should focus on identifying new targets and developing strategies to overcome drug resistance, thereby maximizing the therapeutic potential of this vital approach in combatting parasitic infections globally. A detailed understanding of parasite metabolism, coupled with cutting-edge technologies and a holistic approach to drug development and deployment, is crucial to the continued success of targeting metabolic pathways as an antiparasitic armament.

2.2 Disrupting Reproduction

Targeting parasite reproduction offers a potent strategy in antiparasitic drug development. Interfering with the complex life cycles of these organisms, from asexual multiplication to sexual reproduction and transmission, can effectively disrupt their propagation and reduce infection prevalence. This approach holds immense promise, especially considering the rising challenge of drug resistance. Many parasites exhibit intricate reproductive mechanisms, making them vulnerable to specific interventions. For instance, some rely on specific hormonal signaling pathways for maturation and reproduction; disrupting these pathways could prove highly effective.

Several avenues exist for disrupting parasitic reproduction. One approach involves the development of drugs that interfere with the parasite's ability to produce or utilize essential molecules needed for reproduction, such as specific proteins or nucleic acids. These drugs could target key enzymes involved in DNA replication, RNA transcription, or protein synthesis, effectively halting the parasite's reproductive machinery. This targeted approach minimizes potential damage to the host's cells, improving the overall safety profile of the drug. Another avenue is to develop compounds that prevent the formation of gametes or interfere with fertilization processes. Such compounds could work by blocking the interaction of specific molecules essential for gamete recognition and fusion, or by interfering with the signaling pathways that regulate these processes. This would prevent the parasite from completing its reproductive cycle, effectively controlling its population growth.

The development of antiparasitic drugs targeting reproduction requires a thorough understanding of the parasite's reproductive biology and life cycle. This necessitates detailed research into the molecular mechanisms underpinning the parasite's reproductive processes, identifying key targets for drug intervention. Moreover, understanding the parasite's interactions with its host is vital. The successful development and deployment of such drugs necessitate meticulous research and testing in various models, ensuring efficacy and minimizing adverse effects on the host. This multi-faceted approach is crucial for developing novel therapies that effectively disrupt parasite reproduction without compromising the health of the infected individual. Detailed in vitro and in vivo studies are paramount to validate the efficacy and safety profile of potential compounds.

Furthermore, computational modeling and advanced screening technologies are being employed to accelerate the discovery and optimization of novel compounds targeting reproductive processes. High-throughput screening of large compound libraries allows the rapid identification of potential drug candidates. These candidates are then refined through structure-activity relationship studies, ultimately optimizing their effectiveness and selectivity against target parasite reproductive pathways. Computational modeling helps in predicting the binding affinity of drug candidates to their target sites, which saves time and resources in the drug development pipeline. This advanced approach enables a more efficient and cost-effective identification of potential therapeutics, enabling a faster transition from bench to bedside. Such innovations substantially enhance the chances of successfully developing effective anti-parasitic agents.

Beyond the development of novel drugs, alternative strategies are also being investigated. These include the exploration of existing drugs repurposed for their anti-reproductive effects on parasites. This approach leverages the knowledge already accumulated about the safety and efficacy profiles of these drugs, accelerating the development of new antiparasitic treatments. Careful investigation of their anti-reproductive mechanisms and efficacy against various parasite species is needed. The exploration of natural products as sources of novel anti-reproductive agents is another promising area of research. Many plants and microorganisms synthesize compounds with potent biological activities, some of which may be effective against parasite reproduction. This strategy offers a vast and largely untapped resource for discovering novel compounds that can be developed into effective antiparasitic drugs. Ethnobotanical studies and advanced screening techniques are utilized to identify such potent compounds and subsequently investigate their mechanisms of action.

2.3 Inhibiting Enzyme Activity

Enzyme inhibition forms a cornerstone of many effective antiparasitic strategies. Targeting specific enzymes crucial for parasite survival offers a highly selective approach, minimizing harm to the host. This precision is paramount, given the often delicate balance between eliminating the parasite and preserving the patient's health. Understanding the intricate workings of these enzymes is therefore critical for designing effective and safe treatments.

Several classes of enzyme inhibitors are employed. Competitive inhibitors, for instance, resemble the enzyme's natural substrate and compete for binding at the active site. This competition effectively slows down or blocks the enzyme's catalytic activity. The effectiveness of a competitive inhibitor often depends on its concentration relative to the substrate concentration; higher inhibitor concentrations generally lead to greater inhibition. A clever strategy involves designing inhibitors that exploit the parasite's unique metabolic pathways, ensuring minimal interaction with analogous human enzymes.

Non-competitive inhibitors, in contrast, bind to a site on the enzyme distinct from the active site, altering the enzyme's conformation and reducing its catalytic efficiency. This allosteric binding can either hinder substrate binding or impair the enzyme's catalytic mechanism. The impact of non-competitive inhibitors is less dependent on substrate concentration, making them potentially more effective even at lower concentrations compared to competitive inhibitors. Researchers consistently strive to discover and develop potent non-competitive inhibitors targeting crucial enzymes within parasites.

Uncompetitive inhibitors bind only to the enzyme-substrate complex, thereby preventing the release of products and effectively shutting down the catalytic cycle. This unique mechanism renders them particularly effective against enzymes operating at high substrate concentrations. The design and optimization of such inhibitors require sophisticated understanding of enzyme kinetics and reaction mechanisms.

This intricate interplay of inhibitor binding and enzyme function offers a rich landscape for drug development.

Irreversible inhibitors form covalent bonds with the enzyme, permanently inactivating it. These inhibitors are highly potent, but their permanence also poses challenges in terms of potential side effects. The specificity of the inhibitor is vital to ensure it only targets the parasitic enzyme and not its human counterpart. The development of irreversible inhibitors requires careful consideration of both potency and selectivity. It's a delicate balancing act between achieving maximal effectiveness and minimizing any unintended consequences for the host.

Beyond these general mechanisms, researchers continually explore more nuanced strategies. This includes developing inhibitors that target specific isoforms of enzymes, exploiting differences in enzyme structure between the parasite and the host. This targeted approach maximizes efficacy while minimizing off-target effects. Furthermore, the development of prodrugs–inactive precursors that are converted into active inhibitors within the parasite–offers another avenue for enhancing selectivity and reducing toxicity. This clever approach leverages the parasite's unique intracellular environment to activate the drug specifically within the target.

The rational design of enzyme inhibitors necessitates a deep understanding of enzyme structure and function. Sophisticated techniques like X-ray crystallography and molecular modeling allow scientists to visualize the enzyme's three-dimensional structure and identify potential binding sites for inhibitor molecules. This knowledge is then used to guide the synthesis and optimization of novel inhibitors, allowing for the creation of highly specific and effective drugs. Furthermore, computational methods have become indispensable tools in this process, enabling efficient screening of vast chemical libraries and the prediction of inhibitor efficacy and selectivity. This approach significantly accelerates the drug discovery pipeline.

In addition to traditional small-molecule inhibitors, researchers are exploring other modalities, such as peptide-based inhibitors and antibody-based therapies. Peptide inhibitors mimic natural substrates or regulatory molecules, offering high specificity and potentially reducing side effects. Antibody-based therapies, on the other hand, directly target parasitic enzymes, offering a promising approach, particularly for treating infections caused by parasites that exhibit high levels of drug resistance. These strategies, often involving advanced techniques such as phage display and antibody engineering, represent the forefront of antiparasitic drug development.

The quest for effective antiparasitic drugs hinges on ongoing research into novel enzyme inhibition strategies. This continuous effort to identify and exploit vulnerabilities within parasitic enzymes is essential to combat the ever-evolving challenge of parasitic infections. The development of new inhibitors requires a multidisciplinary approach, incorporating expertise in biochemistry, pharmacology, medicinal chemistry, and computational biology. This collaborative effort is key to delivering safer and more effective treatments, ultimately improving global health outcomes. Each advancement pushes the boundaries of our understanding and capabilities, resulting in improved therapies that offer hope for patients suffering from parasitic diseases worldwide. The ongoing development of new inhibitors is a testament to the relentless pursuit of better healthcare solutions.

3 Drug Resistance & Management

The insidious rise of drug resistance in parasitic infections poses a significant threat to global health. Understanding the mechanisms driving this resistance is paramount to developing effective countermeasures. Parasites, remarkably adaptable organisms, employ various strategies to survive drug exposure. Genetic mutations, altering the drug target site or enhancing drug efflux, are common mechanisms. Changes in drug metabolism, including increased enzyme activity that degrades the drug, also contribute to resistance. Furthermore, parasites may develop alternative metabolic pathways, bypassing the drug's primary mode of action. These complex adaptive processes necessitate a multifaceted approach to management.

Combating drug resistance demands a shift beyond relying solely on single-drug therapies. The use of combination therapies, employing drugs with different mechanisms of action, is crucial. This approach minimizes the likelihood of resistance developing to all drugs simultaneously, reducing the chances of treatment failure. Careful monitoring of parasite drug susceptibility is essential, guiding clinicians in selecting the most effective regimens. Regular surveillance and genomic analysis provide invaluable data on the prevailing resistance patterns within specific geographic areas. This allows for tailoring treatment strategies to target prevalent resistance mechanisms, maximizing efficacy. Moreover, improved diagnostic tools are critical to accurately identifying the parasite species and its resistance profile, enabling prompt and targeted treatment. This reduces unnecessary drug use and minimizes the selection pressure for further resistance development.

Beyond combination therapies, the development of novel antiparasitic drugs is vital. Researchers are actively exploring various strategies, including identifying novel drug targets within parasites and developing drugs that circumvent existing resistance mechanisms. Targeting essential parasite processes that are less prone to mutation or those that differ significantly from human counterparts is a key focus. This approach aims to minimize the chance of cross-resistance and side effects, further improving the effectiveness of these new treatments. The exploration of natural products, often rich in bioactive compounds, provides a vast reservoir of potential drug candidates. These natural sources are frequently investigated for their antiparasitic properties, offering potentially less toxic and effective treatments.

Furthermore, the integration of improved public health measures significantly reduces the emergence and spread of drug resistance. Improving sanitation and hygiene practices minimizes parasitic infections, thus decreasing the selective pressure for drug resistance to evolve. Educational programs focusing on hygiene and preventative measures, especially in endemic regions, are vital in decreasing the overall parasite burden and the need for frequent treatment. Vector control programs play a crucial role in reducing parasite transmission, directly impacting the number of individuals exposed to drugs. Consequently, responsible drug use and the avoidance of unnecessary treatment, while essential in human health, further contribute to limiting the spread of resistance. These measures are not mutually exclusive, but work synergistically in delaying or preventing the development of drug resistance. A comprehensive approach is vital in the continuous fight against the increasing threat of drug resistance in parasitic infections.

The implementation of effective drug resistance management strategies requires a collaborative, multidisciplinary effort. This involves close cooperation between clinicians, researchers, public health officials, and policymakers. Effective surveillance systems are critical for tracking resistance patterns and adapting treatment strategies accordingly. This necessitates standardized data collection and analysis, providing a clear picture of the evolving resistance landscape. Furthermore, strong regulatory frameworks that guide the appropriate use of antiparasitic drugs and monitor their efficacy are essential in preventing the misuse and overuse that fuels resistance. Investment in research and development for new drugs and diagnostic tools is crucial for sustaining the battle against this global health challenge. Finally, international collaborations are necessary to share knowledge, resources, and best practices, working together to address this shared threat effectively. Without this collective effort, the threat of widespread, untreatable parasitic infections remains a grave concern.

3.1 Mechanisms of Resistance

Parasites, masters of adaptation, employ a diverse arsenal of strategies to withstand the onslaught of antiparasitic drugs. Genetic mutations, a cornerstone of resistance, alter the target site of a drug, rendering it ineffective. Imagine a key no longer fitting the lock – the drug can no longer bind and exert its lethal effect. These mutations can arise spontaneously or be selected for under drug pressure, leading to a population of resistant parasites thriving where their susceptible counterparts perish. This is not a passive process; it's a dynamic arms race, a constant push and pull between parasite evolution and drug development.

Another significant mechanism involves altered drug uptake or efflux. Parasites can modify their cell membranes, creating barriers that prevent drugs from entering. Conversely, they might enhance their ability to pump drugs out, effectively reducing the drug's intracellular concentration and minimizing its impact. Think of it as a sophisticated defense system, actively removing the threat before it can cause damage. This active expulsion mechanism is crucial, especially in parasites with high metabolic rates and those inhabiting harsh environments. These adaptations are often encoded in genes, emphasizing the intricate interplay between genetics and the environment.

Beyond these genetic changes, parasites can employ metabolic bypasses to circumvent the drug's action. If a drug inhibits a specific metabolic pathway, the parasite may develop alternative pathways, utilizing different enzymes or substrates to achieve the same outcome. The parasite, cleverly avoiding the drug's target, remains functional and continues to reproduce. This adaptability highlights the parasite's remarkable resilience. This is why a deeper understanding of parasitic metabolic pathways is critical in developing effective treatment strategies.

Environmental factors also play a pivotal role. For example, the presence of other drugs or environmental toxins can interact with the antiparasitic drug, reducing its efficacy or even triggering resistance mechanisms. The interplay between various factors further complicates the picture, underlining the need for a holistic approach to combating resistance. This interaction can be synergistic or antagonistic, further highlighting the complexity of drug resistance.

Furthermore, some parasites exhibit reduced drug susceptibility due to factors such as increased detoxification of the drug or changes in drug activation. These parasites may possess enhanced enzyme systems that degrade or modify the drug, making it less effective. Alternatively, they might alter the process by which the drug becomes active within the parasite's cells, reducing its potency. This process is often less well-understood but significant, particularly in parasites that have been exposed to many drugs over time.

The complexity of parasitic resistance highlights the importance of understanding these multiple and often intertwined mechanisms. Researchers are actively investigating these processes, aiming to develop new strategies to combat drug resistance. This requires a multi-faceted approach, including drug combination therapies, improved diagnostics to identify resistant strains, and the development of novel antiparasitic agents that target different pathways or mechanisms. It's a continuous battle against adaptation and evolution that demands innovative strategies, constant monitoring, and comprehensive analysis to ensure treatment success. The future of antiparasitic therapy hinges on this ongoing research and the integration of new, cutting-edge discoveries. Only through such a concerted effort can we hope to maintain effective control over these highly adaptable organisms.

3.2 Combating Drug Resistance

The insidious rise of drug resistance in parasitic infections poses a significant threat to global health. Understanding the mechanisms driving this resistance is paramount to developing effective countermeasures. We've seen firsthand how parasites, with their remarkable adaptability, can quickly evolve to circumvent the effects of even the most potent drugs. This necessitates a multifaceted approach, moving beyond simply creating new drugs to encompass strategies that actively impede the development of resistance.

One critical strategy focuses on optimizing existing treatments. This isn't about simply increasing dosages—a tactic often counterproductive and potentially harmful. Instead, it involves a meticulous analysis of drug pharmacokinetics and pharmacodynamics within the host and the parasite. Precise dosing regimens, tailored to individual patient characteristics and infection severity, can enhance efficacy and minimize the selective pressure that fuels resistance. This approach is particularly vital in treating chronic infections where continuous drug exposure provides ample opportunity for resistance to develop.

Another key element is improving diagnostic capabilities. Rapid and accurate identification of the parasite species and its susceptibility profile is crucial for guiding treatment decisions. This allows clinicians to select the most effective drugs from the outset, avoiding the use of drugs to which the parasite already exhibits resistance. Advanced molecular diagnostic techniques like PCR-based assays are instrumental in providing this information quickly and reliably, enabling more targeted and effective treatment. Without this precision, we risk accelerating the development of widespread resistance.

Furthermore, we must embrace a paradigm shift in how we approach treatment. The era of single-drug therapies is, in many cases, over. Combining drugs with different mechanisms of action is crucial. This synergistic approach reduces the selective pressure on any single drug, hindering the parasite's ability to develop resistance to the entire regimen. This combination therapy should involve carefully chosen drugs that have minimal overlapping resistance mechanisms. Rigorous research and clinical trials are essential to identifying optimal drug combinations for various parasitic infections.

Beyond drug combinations, exploring alternative therapeutic approaches is vital. This involves investigating new drug targets within the parasite, moving away from those already under selective pressure. Research into novel antiparasitic compounds derived from natural sources, such as plants and microorganisms, is yielding promising results. These compounds often have unique mechanisms of action, offering a fresh avenue for combating resistant parasites. Additionally, innovative drug delivery systems, such as nanoparticles, can improve drug efficacy and reduce toxicity, further enhancing treatment outcomes and minimizing the development of resistance. These newer, smarter strategies offer better outcomes than simply relying on higher doses.

Ultimately, combating drug resistance requires a global, collaborative effort. Surveillance programs, designed to monitor the emergence and spread of resistant parasites, are indispensable for early detection and timely intervention. This information needs to be readily available to clinicians worldwide, enabling them to make informed treatment decisions. International collaborations are critical for sharing data, research findings, and best practices, ensuring a unified approach to this global challenge. A coordinated response, focused on prevention, early detection, and well-defined treatment protocols, offers the best hope of containing the threat of drug-resistant parasites. Only through such a coordinated response can we effectively protect global health.

4 Novel Drug Development

Developing novel antiparasitic drugs necessitates a multi-pronged approach, leveraging cutting-edge technologies and integrating traditional knowledge. Targeted therapies, focusing on specific parasite vulnerabilities, represent a significant advancement. For example, research into kinases unique to parasitic species offers promising avenues for selective drug action, minimizing harm to the host. Identifying and exploiting these specific biochemical pathways is crucial for creating effective and safe treatments. This requires sophisticated techniques, including genomics and proteomics, to pinpoint essential parasite proteins and metabolic processes. The development of specific inhibitors targeting these unique pathways requires rigorous testing and validation, a process often involving high-throughput screening and computational modeling to assess drug-target interactions and predict efficacy. The ultimate goal is to create drugs with improved therapeutic indices, enhancing efficacy while minimizing side effects. Natural product derivatives continue to be a rich source of inspiration for novel drug development. Many traditional remedies, used for centuries in various cultures, hold promising antiparasitic properties. For instance, artemisinin, derived from the sweet wormwood plant, has revolutionized malaria treatment. However, many other plants and microorganisms contain bioactive compounds with potent antiparasitic activity. Researchers are actively exploring these natural sources, utilizing advanced techniques like bioprospecting and combinatorial chemistry to identify, isolate, and modify these compounds to enhance their efficacy and reduce toxicity. The challenge lies in scaling up production and ensuring consistent quality control, often requiring intricate extraction and purification processes. Further, understanding the underlying mechanisms of action of these natural compounds is essential for rational drug design and optimization.

Gene editing technologies, such as CRISPR-Cas9, offer transformative possibilities in antiparasitic drug development. These powerful tools allow for precise modification of parasite genomes, potentially disrupting key genes involved in virulence, drug resistance, or parasite survival. Imagine using gene editing to disable genes essential for parasite replication or to enhance the immune system's ability to recognize and eliminate parasites. This approach, however, presents significant challenges. Delivering gene editing tools effectively to the parasite within the host, while minimizing off-target effects and ensuring genome stability, requires considerable research and development. Ethical considerations are also paramount, especially regarding potential ecological consequences of genetically modified organisms. Careful risk assessments and regulatory frameworks are vital.

Developing effective vaccines against parasitic infections is a long-term goal of considerable importance. Traditional vaccine strategies haven't yielded widespread success against many parasites, owing to their complex life cycles and ability to evade the immune response. However, recent advances in immunology and vaccine technology, including subunit vaccines, DNA vaccines, and mRNA vaccines, are opening new avenues. Understanding the immune responses elicited by parasitic infections and identifying key parasite antigens is crucial for designing effective vaccines. Preclinical studies and clinical trials are essential to assess the safety and efficacy of new vaccine candidates, requiring considerable time and resources. Successful vaccine deployment also requires robust surveillance systems to monitor vaccine effectiveness and adapt strategies as needed.

Combination therapies represent a crucial strategy for combating drug resistance and enhancing treatment efficacy. Using multiple drugs that target different pathways within the parasite prevents the emergence of resistance and maximizes the chances of parasite elimination. However, choosing appropriate drug combinations requires careful consideration of their pharmacokinetic and pharmacodynamic properties, to minimize toxicity and ensure synergistic activity. Furthermore, drug resistance profiles of parasites in different geographic regions must be considered to optimize treatment strategies and prevent the rapid development of resistance to combination therapies. The use of novel drug combinations often requires careful monitoring of patient responses and possible side effects. The goal of this approach is not only to eradicate parasites but also to prevent widespread resistance.

4.1 Targeted Therapies

The development of targeted therapies represents a significant leap forward in combating parasitic infections. Unlike broad-spectrum drugs that may harm the host, targeted therapies focus on specific parasite vulnerabilities, minimizing side effects and enhancing efficacy. This precision approach is particularly crucial given the growing problem of drug resistance. By exploiting unique aspects of parasite biology, these therapies offer a potent strategy to overcome limitations of conventional treatments. For example, research into parasite-specific enzymes and metabolic pathways has yielded remarkable results, leading to the development of novel drugs that effectively inhibit essential functions without impacting the human host.

Identifying and targeting parasite-specific proteins is a core principle of targeted therapy development. For instance, many parasites rely on unique proteins for survival or replication. Drugs designed to inhibit these proteins offer a highly specific approach to parasite elimination. This approach is exemplified by the successful development of drugs targeting crucial enzymes in the parasite's metabolic processes. These enzymes are often different enough from their human counterparts to allow for selective inhibition. Moreover, advancements in proteomics and genomics are now allowing scientists to identify even more parasite-specific targets. This improved understanding facilitates the development of new drugs with enhanced efficacy and reduced toxicity.

Another promising avenue for targeted therapies lies in exploiting the parasite's unique cell structures. Many parasites possess distinct organelles or cellular mechanisms not found in humans, providing attractive targets for drug development. For example, some parasites rely on specific transport systems to import essential nutrients or export waste products. Drugs designed to interfere with these transport systems can effectively starve or poison the parasite. Likewise, unique features of parasite cell membranes or cell walls provide further opportunities for targeted drug delivery systems. These delivery systems can improve drug efficacy by ensuring that the drug reaches its target while minimizing systemic exposure.

The development of drugs that specifically inhibit parasite reproduction is another vital area of targeted therapy. Many parasites reproduce at incredibly high rates, contributing to the rapid spread of infection. Drugs interfering with parasite reproduction, such as those targeting key enzymes involved in DNA replication or cell division, represent a critical strategy to limit infection spread and control disease transmission. These targeted drugs offer the advantage of not only killing existing parasites but also preventing the reproduction of new ones, ultimately impacting parasite populations more effectively.

However, the development of targeted therapies is not without its challenges. Identifying truly specific targets can be difficult, requiring extensive research to distinguish parasite-specific proteins and pathways from their human counterparts. Additionally, parasites can evolve resistance even to highly targeted therapies. To counter this possibility, a combination approach is frequently used. Combining targeted therapies with other drugs or employing multiple drugs targeting different parasite pathways offers a way to minimize the development of drug resistance. This multi-pronged attack makes it harder for parasites to adapt and increases the chances of successful treatment.

Ongoing research strives to overcome these hurdles. Sophisticated screening techniques are helping to identify new drug candidates with improved specificity and efficacy. Computational modeling is also playing an increasingly important role in predicting the potential interactions of drugs with their targets, thus accelerating the drug discovery process and reducing the time and resources required for testing. Moreover, a strong emphasis is being placed on understanding the mechanisms of drug resistance, paving the way for strategies to overcome resistance and ensure the long-term effectiveness of targeted therapies. The future of antiparasitic drug development rests heavily on the continued refinement and expansion of these targeted approaches.

The development of effective targeted therapies relies on a multidisciplinary effort involving parasitologists, pharmacologists, chemists, and bioinformaticians. It requires a holistic understanding of parasite biology, a deep knowledge of drug design and delivery, and a commitment to innovative research strategies. Collaborations across these different fields are essential to translate cutting-edge research into effective treatments that improve global health outcomes and alleviate the burden of parasitic diseases. The ongoing refinement of these approaches, combined with a continued commitment to research, promises a future with more effective and safer treatments for parasitic infections worldwide.

4.2 Natural Product Derivatives

The exploration of natural products as a source of novel antiparasitic agents offers a compelling avenue for drug discovery. Many plants, fungi, and marine organisms produce bioactive compounds with potent antiparasitic activity, representing a vast, largely untapped reservoir of potential therapeutic molecules. These compounds often exhibit unique modes of action, potentially overcoming resistance mechanisms that have rendered existing drugs ineffective. For instance, artemisinin, a sesquiterpene lactone derived from the Artemisia annua plant, has revolutionized malaria treatment, highlighting the significant therapeutic potential of natural product-derived drugs.

However, harnessing the power of natural products requires a multifaceted approach. The initial challenge lies in identifying and isolating the bioactive compounds responsible for the observed antiparasitic activity. This often involves complex extraction and purification techniques, coupled with bioassays to evaluate the efficacy and selectivity of the isolated compounds. High-throughput screening methods are instrumental in identifying promising leads from complex natural product extracts. Furthermore, chemical modification of the lead compounds often enhances their potency, selectivity, and pharmacokinetic properties, crucial for developing effective and safe drugs.

One significant advantage of natural product derivatives is their inherent structural diversity. This translates into a broader range of potential drug targets and mechanisms of action, increasing the likelihood of discovering effective drugs against parasites resistant to conventional therapies. Many natural products target unique parasite pathways not affected by currently available drugs, thereby providing a new strategy to combat drug resistance. For example, some natural products interfere with parasite motility, attachment to host cells, or nutrient uptake, offering alternative targets to those typically addressed by existing antiparasitic agents. Research into the synergistic effects of combining natural product derivatives with conventional drugs is also crucial, potentially enhancing efficacy and delaying the onset of drug resistance.

The development of natural product-derived antiparasitic drugs necessitates rigorous preclinical and clinical evaluation to ensure their safety and efficacy. Toxicity studies are essential to assess potential side effects, while pharmacokinetic and pharmacodynamic studies determine the drug's absorption, distribution, metabolism, and excretion profiles. The clinical development process involves several phases, beginning with small-scale human trials to evaluate safety and tolerability, culminating in large-scale trials to confirm efficacy and determine optimal dosing regimens. This comprehensive testing ensures the development of safe and effective therapies for parasitic infections.

Beyond the scientific challenges, ethical considerations and sustainable sourcing of natural products are critical aspects of drug development. Ensuring ethical harvesting and sustainable management of natural resources protects biodiversity and prevents environmental degradation. Collaboration with local communities and traditional healers can provide valuable insights into the use and efficacy of traditional medicines, facilitating the identification of promising leads. Intellectual property rights associated with natural product-derived drugs also require careful consideration, balancing the interests of researchers, pharmaceutical companies, and local communities. Ultimately, effective collaboration across disciplines is essential for ensuring responsible and sustainable development of antiparasitic drugs derived from nature's rich chemical diversity. The ultimate goal is to translate the therapeutic potential of natural products into safe, efficacious, and accessible treatments for millions affected by parasitic infections worldwide. Such a future requires a sustained commitment to both fundamental and translational research, supported by international collaborations and sustainable resource management practices. Only through such a comprehensive effort can the full potential of natural products be realized to combat the global threat of parasitic diseases.

4.3 Gene Editing Approaches

Gene editing technologies offer a revolutionary approach to combating parasitic infections, addressing the limitations of conventional antiparasitic drugs. CRISPR-Cas9, a particularly promising system, allows for precise targeting and modification of parasitic genomes. This precision is crucial, minimizing off-target effects and enhancing the safety profile of this approach. Imagine being able to precisely disable genes essential for parasite survival, effectively crippling their ability to infect and replicate. This is the power of gene editing.

The application of CRISPR-Cas9 to eliminate or modify genes responsible for drug resistance is particularly exciting. By targeting specific mutations that confer resistance, researchers aim to restore the efficacy of existing antiparasitic drugs, extending their lifespan and improving treatment outcomes. For instance, in Plasmodium falciparum, the parasite responsible for the most severe form of malaria, the gene pfcrt is associated with resistance to chloroquine. Gene editing could theoretically revert this mutation, thus rendering the parasite susceptible again. This targeted approach bypasses the inherent limitations of broad-spectrum antiparasitic drugs and offers a tailored strategy.

Beyond reversing drug resistance, gene editing holds potential for targeting other crucial parasite processes. Imagine incapacitating genes responsible for parasite virulence factors, the molecules that contribute to disease severity. Eliminating these factors could significantly reduce the pathology associated with parasitic infections, leading to milder symptoms and improved patient outcomes. This represents a shift from simply killing the parasite to modulating its disease-causing potential.

However, the challenges in translating gene editing technology from the laboratory to clinical settings are substantial. Delivering the CRISPR-Cas9 machinery effectively to the parasite within the host is a major hurdle. The system needs to be carefully packaged and targeted to reach the parasitic cells without harming the host. Developing efficient delivery vectors, such as modified viruses or nanoparticles, is an active area of research. Furthermore, careful consideration must be given to the potential for off-target effects, which could have unforeseen consequences on the host or the parasite's microbiome. Rigorous testing and validation are essential before clinical application.

Another important consideration is the ethical implications of using gene editing in parasites. The potential for unintended ecological consequences requires careful evaluation. Altering the genetic makeup of parasites could have unforeseen effects on their populations and their interactions with the environment. The development of sophisticated monitoring and risk assessment strategies is crucial to ensure responsible implementation. Discussions involving scientists, ethicists, and policymakers are needed to establish comprehensive ethical guidelines. Furthermore, the cost-effectiveness of gene editing technologies needs to be carefully evaluated. The development and implementation of such techniques can be expensive, potentially limiting their accessibility in resource-limited settings where parasitic infections are most prevalent. Strategies to make gene-editing approaches more affordable and accessible to underserved populations are needed to ensure equitable distribution of this powerful technology. Focusing research on simpler and cost-effective gene editing approaches is important in order to make it accessible to populations across the globe.

Despite these challenges, the potential of gene editing in antiparasitic strategies is undeniable. By combining this revolutionary technology with other innovative approaches, such as drug development and vaccine research, we can create a more comprehensive and effective arsenal to combat parasitic infections. Gene editing offers a new paradigm in parasitology, moving beyond simply treating symptoms to fundamentally altering the parasite's biology. This proactive strategy has the potential to significantly reduce the global burden of parasitic diseases. The future application of this technology holds promise for lasting impact on global health. Continued research and careful consideration of ethical and economic aspects are imperative to fully realize the transformative potential of gene editing in this field. The development and implementation of this approach requires a collaborative effort, bringing together scientists, clinicians, policymakers, and community stakeholders. The ultimate goal is to achieve sustainable and equitable access to this technology to mitigate the substantial global health burden of parasitic diseases.

4.4 Vaccine Development

Developing effective vaccines against parasitic infections presents unique challenges compared to viral or bacterial vaccines. Parasites exhibit complex life cycles, often involving multiple hosts and developmental stages, each potentially requiring a different vaccine strategy. A single vaccine targeting all stages might be incredibly difficult, if not impossible, to achieve. Therefore, focusing on the most vulnerable stages, such as larval forms or the stages associated with disease transmission, represents a more feasible and impactful initial approach.

This complexity extends to the parasites' antigens. Unlike viruses with relatively few surface proteins, parasites present a vast array of antigens, many of which are highly variable due to genetic diversity or antigenic variation mechanisms. This variability poses a significant hurdle for vaccine design, as a vaccine targeting one antigen might prove ineffective against other parasite strains or variants. The development of broad-spectrum vaccines necessitates identifying conserved antigens present across diverse parasite populations, a task demanding sophisticated immunological and genetic analyses. One approach is focusing on antigens associated with essential parasite processes.

Traditional vaccine strategies, primarily focusing on humoral immunity, may not be sufficient for all parasitic infections. Some parasites are able to evade antibody-mediated clearance by mechanisms like antigenic variation or by hiding within host cells. Therefore, a multipronged approach to vaccine development, incorporating cell-mediated immunity through strategies like inducing cytotoxic T lymphocytes (CTLs), is often essential. This strategy could involve recombinant protein vaccines, live attenuated parasites, or DNA vaccines, all designed to stimulate a broader range of immune responses.

Another challenge lies in the delivery of the vaccine. For parasites with complex life cycles, delivery methods need to be tailored to target the relevant life stage. For instance, vaccines targeting the larval stage might be administered orally, while vaccines directed against the adult stage in the blood stream might require parenteral administration. The development of effective delivery systems is crucial for achieving broad efficacy. Moreover, different parasite groups might require entirely different approaches and this is where research on innovative methods like microneedle patches and mucosal delivery systems could prove extremely valuable.

Furthermore, the evaluation of vaccine efficacy is intricate and demands rigorous clinical trials. This complexity is further amplified by the diverse geographical distribution and transmission modes of various parasitic infections. Controlled trials often require careful selection of study populations, consideration of co-infections, and sensitive outcome measures. The establishment of reliable and accurate diagnostic tools for measuring parasite burden and the immune response induced by the vaccine are also paramount.

Despite these challenges, advancements in immunology, molecular biology, and vaccine technology are paving the way for the development of more effective antiparasitic vaccines. The use of advanced technologies like genomics, proteomics, and bioinformatics enables the identification of novel vaccine candidates and the development of improved vaccine formulations. Approaches like reverse vaccinology, which identifies potential vaccine candidates through in silico analysis of parasite genomes, have expedited the process significantly. And the increasing understanding of parasite-host interactions has opened the door for the development of vaccines that target critical mechanisms of pathogenesis.

The future of antiparasitic vaccine development lies in collaborative efforts involving researchers, public health organizations, and pharmaceutical companies. The integration of these expertise is key to addressing the challenges and realizing the potential of vaccines to combat the global burden of parasitic diseases. International collaborations are needed to facilitate the development and distribution of vaccines tailored to specific regions and populations. Finally, sustainable funding mechanisms are vital for the long-term success of this crucial endeavor. Only through continued commitment and a collaborative approach can we overcome the hurdles of antiparasitic vaccine development and make meaningful progress in controlling the widespread impact of these debilitating diseases.

4.5 Combination Therapies

The effectiveness of monotherapy, using a single drug against parasitic infections, is increasingly challenged by the emergence of drug resistance. Parasites, like any living organism, possess remarkable adaptive capabilities, evolving mechanisms to circumvent the lethal effects of specific drugs. This evolutionary pressure drives the selection of resistant strains, rendering previously effective treatments obsolete. This necessitates a paradigm shift towards combination therapies, employing multiple drugs with different mechanisms of action to combat this problem.

A fundamental principle underpinning combination therapy lies in the synergistic effect achieved by using drugs that target different aspects of the parasite's biology. One drug might inhibit a key metabolic pathway, while another might disrupt reproduction or interfere with essential enzyme activity. This multi-pronged approach not only enhances the overall efficacy but also dramatically reduces the likelihood of developing resistance. The parasites are less likely to develop resistance mechanisms that circumvent all drugs simultaneously.

Consider the case of malaria, a devastating parasitic disease affecting millions globally. The rise of artemisinin resistance underscores the critical need for effective combination therapies. Artemisinin-based combination therapies (ACTs), combining artemisinin with another antimalarial drug, are currently the gold standard. This strategy effectively delays or prevents the emergence of resistance, improving treatment outcomes and overall public health. The success of ACTs showcases the power of combination therapies in managing drug-resistant infections.

The judicious selection of drugs for combination therapy is crucial. Factors such as the pharmacokinetic and pharmacodynamic properties of each drug, their potential for interaction, and their safety profiles must be carefully considered. For instance, combining drugs with similar mechanisms of action might not offer significant advantages, while those with overlapping or complementary effects could prove highly synergistic. Careful selection minimizes the risk of adverse effects and ensures optimal treatment efficacy.

Developing new combination therapies involves a complex interplay of scientific disciplines. Parasitologists, pharmacologists, and clinicians collaborate to identify promising drug combinations through in vitro and in vivo studies. This rigorous testing allows researchers to evaluate the efficacy, safety, and synergistic potential of various drug combinations against a range of parasites. Furthermore, preclinical studies are essential to assess drug absorption, distribution, metabolism, and excretion before initiating clinical trials in human populations.

Implementing effective combination therapies requires robust surveillance systems to monitor the emergence and spread of drug resistance. This involves regular monitoring of parasite populations for resistance markers and gathering data on treatment outcomes. This data informs public health policies, ensuring that treatment guidelines are continually updated to reflect evolving drug resistance patterns. The goal is proactive management to maintain treatment efficacy and prevent widespread resistance.

Beyond the scientific advancements, successful implementation of combination therapies demands strong health systems and infrastructure. Access to quality diagnostics, reliable drug supply chains, and trained healthcare professionals are crucial. This is particularly important in resource-limited settings where parasitic infections pose the greatest threat. Ensuring equitable access to effective combination therapies is fundamental to controlling and eliminating parasitic diseases globally.

However, challenges remain in the development and implementation of combination therapies. The cost of developing and manufacturing new drugs can be substantial, posing a significant barrier to access, particularly in low-income countries. The complexities of drug interactions and potential adverse effects need careful consideration. Furthermore, the emergence of resistance to multiple drugs, multi-drug resistance, poses a formidable challenge, necessitating innovative approaches to combat this threat. This might include exploring novel drug targets, repurposing existing drugs, or developing new therapeutic strategies.

In conclusion, combination therapies represent a critical advancement in the fight against parasitic infections. By leveraging the synergistic effects of multiple drugs with different mechanisms of action, these strategies offer significant advantages in combating drug resistance and improving treatment outcomes. However, the successful implementation of these therapies requires ongoing research, robust surveillance systems, and strong healthcare infrastructure to ensure equitable access and prevent the spread of drug resistance. The future of antiparasitic treatment hinges on the continued exploration and development of innovative combination therapies. This requires a comprehensive and coordinated global effort that addresses scientific, economic, and social challenges to ensure that effective treatments reach those most in need. The continuous refinement and expansion of combination therapy strategies will remain central to controlling parasitic diseases and safeguarding global public health. Addressing these challenges will ultimately determine the effectiveness of global antiparasitic efforts.

5 Treatment Modalities: Malaria

The mainstay of malaria treatment remains artemisinin-based combination therapies (ACTs). These combine artemisinin, a fast-acting drug derived from a Chinese herb, with a longer-lasting partner drug like lumefantrine, mefloquine, or amodiaquine. This synergistic approach targets multiple parasite stages, minimizing the risk of resistance development and ensuring a more complete parasite clearance. Careful adherence to the prescribed dosage and treatment duration is crucial for effective treatment and preventing relapse. Monitoring patients for adverse reactions, such as nausea, vomiting, or allergic responses, is essential, and appropriate management strategies should be readily available. The World Health Organization (WHO) provides guidelines on the appropriate ACT regimen depending on the geographical location and prevalent parasite species; staying updated on these recommendations is critical for clinicians. Failure to adhere to these guidelines can lead to treatment failures and the propagation of drug-resistant strains. Therefore, maintaining current knowledge about updated guidelines and recommended dosages for a particular region remains vital in treating malaria successfully.

Beyond ACTs, alternative treatments are explored in cases of resistance or when ACTs are contraindicated. Quinine, a traditional antimalarial, might be used in severe cases or when ACTs are unavailable, although its efficacy is diminished by its relatively high toxicity compared to newer drugs. Other options include atovaquone-proguanil, which is often given as a preventative measure but can also be used for treatment in specific circumstances. However, resistance to these alternatives is emerging, highlighting the pressing need for further research into new antimalarial drugs and treatment strategies. The decision to prescribe alternative treatments should be a careful one made by a qualified healthcare professional, involving a consideration of drug resistance patterns and patient-specific factors such as age, comorbidities, and pregnancy status. The successful implementation of alternative treatment modalities often necessitates a tailored approach to treatment, guided by a thorough understanding of the local epidemiological situation and drug resistance profiles.

Preventing malaria is fundamentally important, given its devastating impact on global health. Vector control measures, primarily targeting the Anopheles mosquito vector, form a crucial aspect of prevention. This involves using insecticide-treated bed nets (ITNs), indoor residual spraying (IRS), and larvicides to reduce mosquito populations. Community-level education campaigns about these methods also remain pivotal in promoting their use, emphasizing their effectiveness in reducing malaria transmission. The importance of environmental sanitation in reducing breeding sites also cannot be overlooked. The effectiveness of these measures is closely linked to community engagement and sustained public health initiatives, necessitating collaborative efforts between governments, healthcare workers, and local communities to ensure widespread adoption and compliance. Furthermore, regular monitoring of mosquito populations is essential to evaluate the effectiveness of vector control strategies and adjust them based on observed trends and resistance development to existing methods.

Prophylactic measures also play a crucial role in preventing malaria, especially in high-risk populations or travelers to malaria-endemic regions. These include antimalarial drugs taken before, during, and after travel to protect against infection. The choice of prophylactic drug depends on various factors, including the specific malaria region being visited, the individual's health status, and potential drug interactions. However, the increasing prevalence of drug-resistant parasites necessitates careful consideration of drug choice, ensuring that effective prophylaxis is maintained against resistant strains. It is also crucial to counsel travelers about potential side effects and necessary precautions, such as safe storage and proper usage of medication, highlighting the importance of understanding the correct usage to ensure effectiveness. Continuous evaluation of the effectiveness of preventative measures is needed, requiring ongoing research into new prophylactic strategies and the monitoring of drug resistance in malaria parasites. This ensures ongoing adaptation to the ever-evolving landscape of malaria prevention.

5.1 Artemisinin-Based Therapies

Artemisinin, a sesquiterpene lactone, derived from the sweet wormwood plant Artemisia annua, revolutionized malaria treatment. Its discovery, initially documented in ancient Chinese texts, was rediscovered and scientifically validated in the 1970s, leading to a significant decrease in malaria-related mortality. The mechanism of action involves the generation of free radicals within the parasite, leading to oxidative stress and ultimately parasite death. This is particularly effective against the asexual blood stages of Plasmodium, the causative agent of malaria. However, it's crucial to understand that artemisinin alone is rarely used due to the rapid emergence of resistance.

The efficacy of artemisinin lies in its rapid action and its ability to clear parasitemia quickly. This characteristic is vital in reducing disease severity and preventing complications like cerebral malaria. However, its use as a monotherapy is strongly discouraged. The development of resistance against artemisinin derivatives, particularly in Southeast Asia, highlights the need for a carefully considered approach to its use. This resistance, often associated with mutations in parasite genes involved in detoxification pathways, underscores the critical importance of adherence to treatment guidelines. Patients must complete their prescribed course to ensure full eradication of the parasite and to minimize the chances of resistance development.

Therefore, artemisinin-based combination therapies (ACTs) represent the current gold standard for malaria treatment. These combinations typically include an artemisinin derivative paired with a longer-acting partner drug, such as lumefantrine, mefloquine, or sulfadoxine-pyrimethamine. This strategy exploits the synergistic effect of the drugs, enhancing their efficacy and delaying the emergence of resistance. The partner drug provides sustained antimalarial activity after the artemisinin component is cleared from the bloodstream. This strategy is critical for preventing parasite recrudescence, which can lead to persistent infection and development of further resistance.

The selection of a specific ACT depends on several factors, including the prevalence of drug resistance in the region, the patient's age and overall health, and the severity of the infection. Careful consideration of these factors, guided by local health guidelines and recommendations from the World Health Organization, is essential for effective treatment. The increasing prevalence of artemisinin resistance necessitates continuous monitoring of parasite susceptibility and adaptation of treatment strategies accordingly. This proactive approach will contribute to containing the spread of artemisinin resistance and safeguarding the efficacy of these life-saving drugs.

Developing new antimalarial drugs remains a critical global health priority. Research into novel drug targets and alternative drug classes is ongoing, focusing on compounds with different mechanisms of action, reducing the likelihood of cross-resistance with existing drugs. Furthermore, innovative drug delivery systems are being explored to improve treatment compliance and drug efficacy, particularly in resource-limited settings. Simultaneously, efforts to develop effective malaria vaccines are intensifying. While no fully effective vaccine is yet available, ongoing clinical trials show promise and the eventual availability of a vaccine could greatly reduce malaria incidence, consequently decreasing the selective pressure that promotes drug resistance.

Beyond pharmaceutical interventions, vector control remains a cornerstone of malaria prevention and control. Strategies like insecticide-treated bed nets, indoor residual spraying, and larval control significantly reduce mosquito populations, thereby lowering malaria transmission rates. These strategies should be integrated with effective case management to implement comprehensive malaria control programs. Furthermore, community engagement and health education are vital to ensure adherence to preventative measures and early detection of infections. This community-driven approach helps break the transmission cycle and promotes a more sustainable malaria control strategy. The fight against malaria requires a multi-pronged approach that seamlessly combines effective treatment strategies, proactive preventive measures, and robust research efforts to ensure long-term efficacy and public health security. Understanding the complex interplay of these factors is crucial for successful implementation of sustainable and effective malaria control programs.

5.2 Alternative Treatments

Malaria's complexity necessitates exploring options beyond standard artemisinin-based combination therapies (ACTs). These alternative treatments, while not always first-line, play a vital role in managing resistance and addressing specific patient needs. Their efficacy often depends on the parasite strain, the patient's immune status, and the severity of the infection. Careful consideration of these factors is crucial for successful implementation.

Certain herbal remedies have shown some promise in preclinical studies, though rigorous clinical trials are often lacking. For instance, extracts from plants like Artemisia annua, while containing artemisinin precursors, might offer unique compounds with different mechanisms of action. However, standardization of these extracts, ensuring consistent potency and purity, remains a major hurdle. The inherent variability in herbal preparations presents significant challenges for consistent treatment outcomes. Further research, focusing on phytochemical profiling and rigorous clinical evaluation, is essential before widespread adoption can be recommended. It's imperative to avoid unsubstantiated claims and prioritize evidence-based approaches.

Another avenue involves repurposing existing drugs. Some medications, initially developed for other conditions, have shown antimalarial activity in vitro or in animal models. This strategy offers a faster pathway to clinical trials, potentially bypassing the lengthy and expensive process of developing new drugs from scratch. However, careful evaluation of potential drug interactions and toxicity profiles is paramount to ensure patient safety. Repurposing drugs requires extensive pharmacokinetic and pharmacodynamic studies to determine optimal dosages and treatment schedules. The process is complex and demands thorough investigations to identify any unexpected side effects or complications.

In specific situations, supportive care becomes a crucial component of malaria management. This encompasses managing symptoms like fever, dehydration, and anemia. Prompt treatment of complications, such as cerebral malaria, is critical, often requiring intensive care management. For individuals with severe malaria, appropriate supportive care measures can significantly impact overall prognosis, potentially even determining life or death. The integration of supportive care with pharmacological interventions is essential for holistic management of this potentially deadly infection. Access to essential medical resources, including intravenous fluids, blood transfusions, and respiratory support, is vital, particularly in resource-limited settings.

Furthermore, the development of next-generation antimalarial drugs is an ongoing endeavor. Research efforts focus on novel drug targets within the malaria parasite, aiming to overcome existing resistance mechanisms. This involves investigating various pathways vital for parasite survival, such as protein synthesis, DNA replication, and heme biosynthesis. The ultimate goal is the development of highly effective and well-tolerated medications that can be used in combination therapies to prevent the emergence of resistance. This research is complex and requires substantial investment in advanced research technologies and collaborative efforts among scientists and pharmaceutical companies. The process may take many years, but this is an imperative step in combatting malaria's persistent threat.

Finally, strengthening malaria prevention programs, encompassing vector control and improved access to prophylaxis, remains critical. These preventative strategies, though not directly "treatments," are vital in reducing malaria transmission and therefore the overall disease burden. Education regarding personal protective measures, coupled with broad-scale interventions like insecticide-treated bed nets and community-based vector control programs, is essential. Long-term success in battling malaria relies heavily on a multi-pronged approach, encompassing both treatment and robust prevention strategies. Such efforts require global cooperation, significant investment, and sustained commitment to achieve meaningful and lasting impact on public health. The complexity and evolving nature of malaria necessitate a constant re-evaluation of treatment strategies and sustained commitment to research and development.

5.3 Malaria Prevention

Effective malaria prevention hinges on a multi-pronged approach, combining individual protective measures with broader public health interventions. Personal protection relies heavily on minimizing exposure to mosquito bites, the primary vector for malaria transmission. This involves using insecticide-treated bed nets, particularly during peak mosquito biting hours, typically dusk and dawn. Long-sleeved shirts and long trousers, especially in areas with high malaria transmission, provide an additional layer of protection. Repellents containing DEET or other effective ingredients should be applied liberally to exposed skin, following product instructions carefully for optimal safety and efficacy. These strategies work best in combination; relying solely on one method drastically reduces the effectiveness of malaria prevention.

Furthermore, understanding the local malaria transmission patterns is crucial. Knowing the peak mosquito activity periods in a specific region allows for more targeted use of preventative measures. For example, if biting is most intense during the early evening, focusing personal protection efforts around that time will be much more effective than a general all-day approach. Similarly, awareness of high-risk areas within a community or region enables better planning and allocation of resources for mosquito control efforts. This information can be obtained from local health authorities or through research studies on malaria epidemiology in the area. This targeted approach is far more effective than implementing blanket measures indiscriminately.

Beyond individual protection, environmental modification plays a vital role in disrupting malaria transmission. This includes efforts to reduce mosquito breeding sites, such as eliminating stagnant water sources in and around homes and communities. This could involve clearing clogged drains, regularly emptying containers holding water, and maintaining proper drainage systems. Community participation is essential for these types of widespread environmental interventions. Successful implementation relies on educating and engaging the community on the importance of such actions, and ensuring their active involvement in mosquito control efforts.

Public health initiatives can significantly enhance malaria prevention. These include large-scale insecticide spraying programs, carefully targeting mosquito breeding grounds and resting sites. The type of insecticide and frequency of spraying would need to be adapted based on local mosquito species and resistance patterns, requiring continuous monitoring and adjustment. Moreover, indoor residual spraying (IRS), which applies insecticides to the interior walls of houses to kill mosquitoes upon contact, can greatly decrease malaria transmission. However, IRS programs must be carefully implemented, accounting for insecticide resistance and potential health impacts on humans and the environment. Effective public health interventions require careful planning, collaboration with local communities, and sustained monitoring and evaluation.

Finally, the role of chemoprophylaxis, or the use of antimalarial drugs to prevent infection, cannot be overlooked. These medications are available for both short-term use, often for travelers visiting malaria-endemic regions, and long-term use, primarily for individuals living in high-risk areas. The choice of medication and the duration of treatment will depend on factors such as the individual's travel or residence history, age, health status, and the prevalence of drug resistance in the region. Careful consideration of potential side effects and drug interactions is also crucial for safe and effective chemoprophylaxis. Regular consultations with healthcare professionals are essential to ensure appropriate drug selection and monitoring of potential adverse effects. A proactive, informed approach, combining personal protective strategies with robust community and public health interventions and carefully considered chemoprophylaxis, is the cornerstone of successful malaria prevention.

6 Treatment Modalities: Helminths

Helminth infections, encompassing a broad spectrum of parasitic worms, necessitate a multifaceted approach to treatment. Effective management hinges on accurate diagnosis, appropriate drug selection, and consideration of patient-specific factors. Ignoring these nuances can lead to treatment failure and the potential development of drug resistance, highlighting the complexity of managing these infections. The key, therefore, lies in careful consideration of multiple factors. Several anthelmintic drug classes target different aspects of helminth biology. Benzimidazoles, for instance, disrupt microtubule function, impacting the parasites' ability to absorb nutrients and reproduce. Avermectins, derived from soil bacteria, enhance the permeability of helminth cell membranes, leading to their paralysis and eventual death. Pyrantel pamoate, another commonly used anthelmintic, acts as a neuromuscular blocker, causing paralysis and expulsion of the worms. Each drug class has its own spectrum of activity and potential side effects. Precise selection is paramount for optimal therapeutic outcomes.

Treatment strategies must consider the specific helminth species involved. Different worms exhibit varying susceptibility to anthelmintics. For example, Ascaris lumbricoides (roundworm) responds well to albendazole, while Schistosoma mansoni (blood fluke) requires praziquantel for effective treatment. Furthermore, geographical location significantly impacts treatment choices. Variations in prevalent helminth species and the potential for drug resistance necessitate regionally tailored therapeutic approaches. Ignoring these factors can be detrimental to patient outcomes.

Patient age and overall health also influence treatment decisions. Children, for example, may require adjusted dosages compared to adults to minimize potential side effects. Patients with compromised immune systems might experience a more challenging course of infection, and treatment strategies may need to incorporate supportive measures alongside anthelmintic therapy. This highlights the intricate balance between parasite eradication and patient well-being. The approach must always be personalized.

The rise of drug resistance in helminths underscores the need for prudent anthelmintic usage. Overuse and improper administration contribute to this problem, leading to treatment failures and reduced efficacy. Rational drug use, including adherence to prescribed dosages and treatment regimens, is crucial to preserving the effectiveness of existing anthelmintics. Promoting responsible drug use practices, coupled with effective monitoring, should be a priority to avoid the emergence of widespread resistance. The consequences of resistance can be catastrophic.

Combating drug resistance requires a multifaceted approach, extending beyond individual patient treatment. This includes improved diagnostic tools to enable accurate species identification and susceptibility testing. It also necessitates the development of novel anthelmintic drugs targeting different biological pathways and less susceptible to resistance mechanisms. Research into alternative treatment strategies, such as vaccines or immunotherapy, may eventually offer additional options.

Finally, successful helminth treatment necessitates a holistic perspective. Sanitation improvements, hygiene promotion, and public health interventions play a vital role in preventing reinfection. Addressing socioeconomic factors that contribute to parasitic disease transmission is crucial for long-term control and eradication efforts. Treatment success is not just about the medication; it's about addressing all aspects that contribute to the cycle of infection. The broader context, therefore, is crucial. Only by considering all of these elements can we effectively tackle the immense challenge posed by helminth infections globally.

6.1 Anthelmintic Drug Classes

Anthelmintic drugs represent a diverse arsenal in combating helminth infections. Their efficacy hinges on understanding their varied mechanisms of action, which allow for targeted treatment strategies. Benzimidazoles, for instance, disrupt microtubule function within the parasite, inhibiting their energy production and ultimately leading to paralysis and death. This class includes albendazole and mebendazole, widely used against nematodes and cestodes. Their broad-spectrum activity makes them a cornerstone of many treatment regimens, particularly in regions with high helminth prevalence. However, their effectiveness can be compromised by factors such as drug absorption and parasite metabolism, influencing dose selection and treatment duration.

The macrocyclic lactones, including ivermectin and moxidectin, function differently. They bind to glutamate-gated chloride channels in parasite nerve and muscle cells, causing hyperpolarization and paralysis. This class offers excellent efficacy against nematodes, with ivermectin often being the drug of choice for onchocerciasis and lymphatic filariasis, two debilitating diseases affecting millions globally. Moxidectin, with its extended duration of action, offers advantages in treating certain infections, particularly in livestock, although its use in humans is more limited due to ongoing research and safety considerations. Understanding the specific pharmacology and pharmacokinetics of each drug within this class is paramount for effective treatment.

Another crucial class comprises the pyrazinoisoquinolines, exemplified by praziquantel. This drug alters the permeability of the parasite cell membrane, leading to calcium influx and ultimately causing paralysis and death. Its primary target is trematodes and cestodes, making it indispensable in treating schistosomiasis and other fluke infections. Praziquantel's effectiveness depends on the parasite's life cycle stage and the specific species involved. Appropriate dosage and treatment duration are vital for optimal efficacy, considerations influenced by factors such as the patient's age, weight, and the severity of infection. Understanding the specific parasitic species infecting the patient informs praziquantel's optimal deployment.

Additionally, nicotinic agonists like levamisole and pyrantel pamoate, target cholinergic receptors, causing paralysis and expulsion of the parasite. Levamisole, with its immune-modulatory properties, shows efficacy against nematodes. Pyrantel pamoate, similarly, finds wide use as an anthelmintic, particularly in veterinary medicine. However, both drugs may have limitations regarding spectrum of activity and efficacy compared to newer anthelmintics. Their use often hinges on the specific type of nematode infection and consideration of potential side effects and drug interactions.

The choice of anthelmintic drug must consider several critical factors. The specific helminth species, the infection's severity, the patient's age and overall health, and potential drug interactions all play crucial roles. Treatment guidelines, constantly evolving with emerging research, offer essential guidance for clinicians in selecting the optimal anthelmintic drug for a given scenario. Moreover, regional variations in helminth prevalence and drug resistance patterns necessitate adapting treatment strategies to local epidemiological context. The successful treatment hinges on the appropriate drug selection, accurate diagnosis, and a full appreciation of the potential side effects associated with each medication.

Beyond these primary drug classes, several other compounds exhibit anthelmintic activity. These include compounds under investigation for improved efficacy and reduced side effects, such as the piperazine derivatives. Furthermore, advancements in drug delivery systems, aimed at improving bioavailability and reducing toxicity, continue to shape the landscape of anthelmintic therapy. These innovations are particularly relevant in addressing challenges like drug resistance and ensuring treatment reaches remote populations. Understanding the complexities of anthelmintic drug action and adapting treatment strategies to the local context are vital to the ongoing struggle against helminth infections. The continued development of new and improved anthelmintics remains a high priority in global health. Careful consideration of existing treatments is crucial to ensuring successful parasite control globally.

6.2 Treatment Strategies

Effective helminth treatment hinges on accurate diagnosis, a crucial first step often overlooked. Identifying the specific parasite species is paramount; treatment varies significantly depending on whether the infection involves Ascaris lumbricoides, Trichuris trichiura, hookworms, or other species. Misdiagnosis can lead to ineffective therapy, prolonged infection, and potentially severe complications. Therefore, meticulous stool examinations, often complemented by serological tests or imaging techniques like ultrasound, are indispensable. Remember, the choice of anthelmintic depends not only on the infecting species but also on the patient's age, overall health status, and potential drug interactions. Treating pregnant or breastfeeding women, or individuals with compromised immune systems, requires careful consideration and may necessitate alternative treatment strategies.

Beyond species identification, considering the patient's geographic location is equally important. Certain helminth species exhibit geographic clustering, and prevalence varies significantly across regions. Knowledge of local parasite epidemiology guides treatment selection. For instance, drug resistance patterns differ geographically; a drug highly effective in one region might prove ineffective in another due to prevalent resistant strains. This necessitates a nuanced approach, possibly involving resistance testing when feasible. Access to resources, including diagnostic tools and medications, also varies considerably. Therefore, treatment strategies need to be adaptable to diverse contexts, taking into account resource availability and local health system capacity.

The choice of anthelmintic itself presents a range of options, each with distinct advantages and disadvantages. Broad-spectrum drugs, such as albendazole and mebendazole, are frequently used due to their effectiveness against multiple helminth species. However, their efficacy against certain species might be limited, and resistance is an increasing concern. Consequently, the increasing prevalence of resistance necessitates a shift toward targeted therapies whenever possible. These newer agents offer superior efficacy against specific parasites while potentially minimizing side effects and reducing the risk of selecting for drug-resistant strains. However, these newer drugs are often more costly and may not be readily available in all settings.

Treatment regimens often involve a single dose for certain infections, while others require multiple doses over several days or weeks. The optimal duration of treatment depends on several factors, including the parasite's lifecycle, the severity of the infection, and the chosen anthelmintic. In mass drug administration programs, aimed at controlling the prevalence of helminth infections within a population, single-dose treatments are preferred due to logistical simplicity. Individualized treatment, however, demands a more tailored approach, often extending treatment duration to ensure complete parasite eradication and minimize the risk of relapse. Regular follow-up examinations are essential to assess treatment efficacy and detect potential re-infections. This close monitoring is particularly critical in areas with high parasite transmission rates.

Beyond medication, there are crucial non-pharmacological interventions. Improved sanitation and hygiene practices significantly reduce the risk of re-infection. Educational programs aimed at raising awareness about hygiene and sanitation are integral to successful helminth control. Addressing underlying socioeconomic factors, such as poverty and inadequate access to clean water and sanitation facilities, plays a vital role in long-term helminth control. These factors directly influence the risk of infection and the success of treatment interventions. These holistic approaches, integrating pharmaceutical interventions with public health strategies, are necessary for effective and sustainable helminth control and the prevention of future infections. This necessitates strong interdisciplinary collaboration across medicine, public health, and community engagement to achieve impactful long-term success. It's a complex interplay requiring a multifaceted strategy.

7 Future Directions & Challenges

The escalating global burden of parasitic diseases necessitates a paradigm shift in our approach to control and eradication. Simply developing new drugs isn't enough; we need to consider the complex interplay between human, animal, and environmental health–a true One Health approach. This requires interdisciplinary collaborations, involving parasitologists, pharmacologists, veterinarians, ecologists, and public health officials, to understand the transmission dynamics and implement effective interventions across diverse ecosystems. Ignoring the interconnectedness of these systems will only lead to setbacks in our fight against parasites. Effective surveillance systems, robust diagnostic tools, and community engagement are crucial for successful implementation of One Health strategies.

Successfully tackling parasitic diseases also demands significant investment in research. Prioritizing research on novel drug targets, developing rapid diagnostic tests, and exploring the potential of immunotherapeutic approaches are vital. Understanding the genetic basis of drug resistance is paramount for designing drugs that overcome these mechanisms. We need to foster collaborations between academic institutions, pharmaceutical companies, and funding agencies to ensure that research efforts are impactful and efficiently translated into tangible benefits. Furthermore, exploring the potential of repurposing existing drugs for new parasitic indications could significantly expedite the development process and reduce costs.

The economic impact of parasitic diseases is substantial, affecting both individuals and national economies. The costs associated with treatment, loss of productivity, and the overall burden on healthcare systems are staggering. We must therefore advocate for policies that prioritize access to affordable and effective antiparasitic drugs. This includes strengthening healthcare infrastructure in resource-limited settings and implementing strategies for equitable distribution of treatment. Economic models that account for the long-term costs and benefits of interventions are essential for informed decision-making. Sustainable financing mechanisms and international collaborations are needed to address the economic burden of these diseases effectively.

Efficient and targeted drug delivery remains a significant hurdle, particularly in remote and underserved areas. Developing innovative drug delivery systems tailored to specific parasite life cycles and transmission routes is essential. This includes exploring the potential of nanotechnology-based drug delivery, which could enhance drug efficacy and reduce side effects. Furthermore, improving existing drug formulations to enhance stability and shelf life, especially in tropical climates, is crucial for ensuring accessibility. Addressing these challenges requires collaboration between pharmaceutical scientists and engineers, alongside consideration of the logistical realities of drug distribution in affected regions.

Addressing the challenges posed by parasitic diseases demands a multifaceted approach that goes beyond simply developing new drugs. It involves strengthening healthcare systems, empowering communities, fostering research and development, and implementing effective public health interventions. A commitment to a One Health perspective, coupled with equitable access to affordable treatment and innovative drug delivery systems, is essential for achieving significant progress in the fight against these often neglected diseases. The global community must recognize the interconnectedness of human, animal, and environmental health and work together to address these complex challenges, ensuring a healthier future for all. Only through a collaborative and comprehensive approach can we effectively control and eradicate the devastating impact of parasitic diseases worldwide. The task is ambitious, demanding sustained commitment and innovative strategies across multiple sectors, but the potential rewards – improved global health and economic stability – make this a critical endeavor for our time. The future of antiparasitic armaments depends on our collective willingness to rise to this challenge.

7.1 One Health Approach

The escalating threat of parasitic diseases necessitates a paradigm shift in our approach to treatment and prevention. We can no longer afford to view these infections solely through a human-centric lens. A One Health approach, emphasizing the interconnectedness of human, animal, and environmental health, is crucial for effective and sustainable control. This holistic strategy recognizes that parasites often circulate within complex ecological systems, with spillover events between species contributing significantly to outbreaks. Ignoring the animal reservoir or environmental factors that influence parasite transmission renders any intervention ultimately ineffective. For example, understanding the role of livestock in harboring and transmitting parasites to humans informs strategic interventions targeting both human and animal populations.

Effective implementation requires a multidisciplinary collaboration that transcends traditional sectoral boundaries. Veterinarians, epidemiologists, zoologists, ecologists, and public health officials must work together, sharing data, expertise, and resources. This coordinated effort facilitates more comprehensive surveillance systems, enabling the early detection of emerging parasitic threats and informing rapid, targeted interventions. Furthermore, a One Health approach demands a deeper understanding of the environmental drivers of parasite transmission. Climate change, deforestation, and urbanization all influence parasite distribution and prevalence, creating new challenges that require innovative solutions. Integrating these ecological aspects into our strategies is essential for long-term success.

Consider the example of zoonotic parasitic diseases. These infections spread between animals and humans, highlighting the interconnectedness of our health with that of the animal kingdom. By monitoring parasite prevalence in animal populations, we can anticipate potential spillover events and implement preventive measures. This proactive approach could involve vaccinating animals, improving sanitation practices in animal husbandry, and educating communities about safe handling of animals. Moreover, tackling environmental issues impacting parasite transmission is equally crucial. Improving water sanitation, controlling vector populations, and reducing human exposure to contaminated environments directly contribute to reducing the overall parasite burden. This includes promoting sustainable agricultural practices that minimize environmental contamination and limit the use of pesticides that may have unintended consequences on parasite life cycles and their reservoirs.

This integrated strategy requires significant investments in research and infrastructure. We need advanced diagnostic tools capable of detecting parasites rapidly and accurately, both in humans and animals. This improved diagnostic capacity enables timely interventions and contributes to a more accurate assessment of parasite prevalence. Likewise, investment in research into new antiparasitic drugs, specifically those targeting multiple species or life stages of parasites, is vital to overcome the challenge of drug resistance. This includes exploring novel drug delivery systems that improve efficacy and minimize side effects. Collaboration between research institutions, pharmaceutical companies, and governmental agencies is paramount in accelerating the pace of drug discovery and development. It is also essential to enhance our understanding of the genetic diversity within parasite populations. Genetic characterization allows for a more nuanced understanding of parasite evolution, drug resistance, and transmission dynamics. This improved understanding will ultimately lead to more effective and targeted control strategies.

Furthermore, a One Health approach necessitates strong community engagement. Public health education campaigns play a vital role in fostering awareness and promoting preventive behaviors. This collaborative approach ensures that interventions are culturally appropriate and effectively reach the target populations. Community participation is not merely desirable; it is fundamental to the success of any One Health initiative. Only through collaborative efforts, informed decision-making, and ongoing monitoring can we effectively address the complex challenges posed by parasitic diseases. The global scale of this challenge requires a global response. International collaboration among nations is crucial for sharing knowledge, resources, and best practices, especially in regions with limited resources and infrastructure. A One Health approach is not merely a strategy; it is a philosophical shift, a commitment to a more holistic and sustainable approach to global health security.

7.2 Global Health Initiatives

Global health initiatives play a crucial role in combating parasitic diseases, a significant global health challenge. These initiatives are not simply charitable endeavors; they represent a coordinated, multi-pronged approach requiring substantial investment and collaboration across international borders and diverse disciplines. Successful initiatives demand a comprehensive strategy that addresses the complex interplay of socioeconomic factors, infrastructure limitations, and the inherent biological challenges posed by parasites. Effective implementation necessitates a clear understanding of the disease burden, encompassing not only prevalence and mortality statistics but also the long-term socioeconomic consequences for affected communities.

The World Health Organization (WHO), for instance, spearheads several vital initiatives, providing technical guidance, coordinating research efforts, and facilitating access to essential medicines and diagnostics. However, WHO's effectiveness heavily depends on the financial and logistical support provided by member states and international development organizations, highlighting the complex web of funding and political considerations inherent in global health initiatives. Their success isn't solely measured by drug discovery and distribution but also by community engagement, education programs targeted at prevention, and robust surveillance systems that track emerging parasitic threats. Sustainable funding models are crucial to ensure long-term impact and the avoidance of project-specific funding cycles that often hinder continuity.

Effective global health initiatives must adopt a One Health approach. This holistic framework recognizes the interconnectedness of human, animal, and environmental health. Addressing parasitic diseases requires coordinated efforts across veterinary medicine, public health, and environmental science. This integrated approach is paramount, as many parasites have complex life cycles involving multiple hosts and vectors, such as mosquitoes in malaria or snails in schistosomiasis. Therefore, strategies must not only target the parasite itself but also control vector populations and improve sanitation, thereby interrupting the parasite's transmission cycle.

Developing sustainable capacity within affected countries is equally crucial. Instead of solely relying on external expertise and resources, initiatives should prioritize training local healthcare professionals, building robust healthcare infrastructure, and empowering communities to participate actively in disease prevention and control. This capacity building goes beyond just providing medical training; it also requires investment in laboratory infrastructure, diagnostic capabilities, and data management systems. Furthermore, fostering local research capacity allows for more tailored responses to regional parasite strains and treatment challenges.

A substantial challenge in global health initiatives is ensuring equitable access to effective treatments and preventative measures. Cost-effectiveness considerations must be balanced with the need to make these interventions available to all who need them. This might involve negotiating lower drug prices with pharmaceutical companies, developing affordable generic alternatives, or implementing subsidies and aid programs to ensure affordability and reach in resource-limited settings. Innovative drug delivery strategies, like using point-of-care diagnostics and simpler, more stable drug formulations, must be explored to improve access in remote or underserved areas. This requires a nuanced approach that prioritizes equity and recognizes the unique challenges faced by different communities.

Finally, success hinges on robust monitoring and evaluation frameworks. Regular assessment of initiative effectiveness allows for adaptive management and adjustments based on real-world outcomes. This involves collecting comprehensive data on disease prevalence, treatment outcomes, and the impact of various interventions, which can then inform policy adjustments and resource allocation. Transparency and data sharing are essential to build trust among stakeholders and ensure accountability. Open access to data enables a greater understanding of what works and what doesn't, furthering advancements in the field and ultimately enhancing the efficiency and effectiveness of future initiatives. Ultimately, tackling global parasitic diseases requires a sustained, collaborative, and adaptable global effort.

7.3 Research Priorities

Developing effective and affordable antiparasitic drugs demands a multi-pronged research strategy. Prioritizing research into novel drug targets, particularly those less susceptible to resistance mechanisms, is crucial. This includes exploring unique metabolic pathways, essential for parasite survival but absent in humans, minimizing off-target effects and toxicity. For instance, research into parasite-specific enzymes or proteins involved in crucial processes like nutrient uptake or signal transduction holds immense potential.

A renewed focus on natural product drug discovery is also vital. Many traditional medicines have demonstrated antiparasitic activity, offering a rich source of potential drug leads. However, the challenge lies in isolating the active compounds, determining their mechanisms of action, and developing them into safe and effective drugs. Careful chemical modification of these natural products could enhance their potency and bioavailability, and reduce toxicity.

Furthermore, we must leverage advancements in genomics and proteomics. Comparative genomics can identify genetic differences between parasites and their hosts, providing opportunities for developing highly specific drugs with minimal side effects. Proteomics studies can identify unique parasite proteins that could serve as drug targets, enabling the development of highly targeted therapies.

Combating drug resistance requires a multifaceted approach extending beyond simply developing new drugs. Research into diagnostic tools that rapidly identify drug-resistant parasites is critical for guiding treatment decisions and preventing the spread of resistance. This includes improving molecular diagnostic assays to detect specific resistance markers, facilitating targeted treatment.

Research into innovative drug delivery systems is also essential. Many existing antiparasitic drugs suffer from poor bioavailability, requiring high doses to achieve therapeutic effects. Novel delivery systems, such as nanoparticles or liposomes, could improve drug delivery to the site of infection, increasing efficacy while decreasing toxicity. Such approaches require careful consideration of the pharmacokinetic and pharmacodynamic properties of the drug-delivery system in the context of the specific parasite and host.

A deeper understanding of parasite biology and host-parasite interactions is paramount. This includes investigating the intricate mechanisms by which parasites evade the host's immune system and establish chronic infections. Elucidating these mechanisms is key to designing interventions that enhance host immunity or interfere with parasite survival strategies. This demands sophisticated immunological and molecular biological techniques.

The development of effective vaccines against parasitic infections remains a major challenge. Research into vaccine candidates targeting multiple parasite stages or using novel adjuvants to enhance immune responses is needed. Such research must consider the complexity of parasite life cycles and their ability to evade immune responses and address the significant challenges associated with vaccine development and global implementation.

Finally, a One Health approach should underpin all research efforts. Parasites often circulate between humans, animals, and the environment, requiring a collaborative, interdisciplinary approach. This includes veterinary parasitologists, ecologists, and epidemiologists to effectively tackle parasitic infections. Collaborations between research institutions and pharmaceutical companies are vital to translate research findings into tangible therapeutic benefits. Such synergistic efforts will provide crucial insights into the transmission dynamics of parasitic diseases and pave the way for more effective control strategies. Ultimately, this collaborative approach, underpinned by the research priorities outlined, is essential to combat the devastating impact of parasitic infections globally.

7.4 Challenges in Drug Delivery

Effective drug delivery remains a significant hurdle in combating parasitic infections. Many antiparasitic drugs, while potent in vitro, struggle to reach therapeutic concentrations at the site of infection within the host. This is especially true for parasites residing within protected environments like the liver, brain, or within cysts. For example, achieving sufficient drug levels in the cerebrospinal fluid to treat neurocysticercosis, a parasitic infection of the brain caused by Taenia solium, presents a major challenge, often necessitating the use of high doses with associated toxicities. This highlights the need for innovative drug delivery systems capable of overcoming these barriers.

The physicochemical properties of many antiparasitic drugs further complicate their delivery. Some are poorly soluble in aqueous solutions, limiting their bioavailability and absorption. Others are rapidly metabolized or excreted, reducing their efficacy and requiring frequent administrations, impacting patient compliance. For instance, the poor solubility of some artemisinin derivatives necessitates the use of formulations that enhance solubility and bioavailability, sometimes leading to complex and costly drug products. This issue emphasizes the need to optimize the pharmacokinetic properties of antiparasitic drugs to improve their delivery and efficacy.

Targeting specific organs or tissues is another key challenge. Systemic administration of antiparasitic drugs often leads to off-target effects and toxicity in the host, as the drug affects the entire body. Developing targeted drug delivery systems that can specifically deliver the drug to the site of infection while minimizing systemic exposure is crucial to reduce side effects. One promising approach is the use of nanoparticles that can encapsulate the drug and target specific parasite antigens or host cells, allowing for highly localized drug delivery. However, the development and production of such targeted systems often involves complex and expensive processes. Therefore, the development and scaling up of these targeted delivery systems, while challenging, is crucial to improving patient care and outcomes.

Beyond technological hurdles, socioeconomic factors significantly influence successful drug delivery. Many parasitic infections predominantly affect resource-limited settings, where access to sophisticated drug delivery technologies or even basic healthcare infrastructure may be limited. The logistical challenges of storing, transporting, and administering complex drug delivery systems in these settings must be addressed. For example, the cold-chain requirements for some vaccines and temperature-sensitive antiparasitic drugs pose significant hurdles in areas with unreliable electricity or inadequate refrigeration facilities. Innovative solutions are needed for overcoming these limitations–developing formulations that are stable at ambient temperatures or using simplified delivery methods that are accessible to healthcare workers with minimal training.

Finally, the complex life cycles of many parasites present further complexities for drug delivery. Some parasites have multiple life stages, each with distinct vulnerabilities and locations within the host. To effectively eradicate the parasite, the drug must reach and target all relevant life stages. For instance, the complex life cycle of Plasmodium falciparum, the causative agent of malaria, requires multiple drug administrations to target different stages of the parasite's development in the human host and the mosquito vector. In such cases, combination therapies using drugs with different mechanisms of action and targeting different stages of parasite development are often needed, further complicating delivery strategies. This highlights the need to consider the parasite's life cycle when designing and implementing drug delivery systems to ensure effective treatment. Overcoming these challenges, both technological and logistical, will be essential for developing effective and equitable treatments for parasitic infections worldwide.

7.5 Economic Considerations

The economic burden of parasitic diseases is substantial, impacting both individual households and national economies. Treatment costs, lost productivity due to illness and disability, and the expense of preventative measures all contribute to a significant financial strain. For individuals, particularly in low-income countries, the cost of medication, hospital visits, and potential loss of income can be catastrophic, pushing families further into poverty and hindering their ability to escape the cycle of infection. This is especially true for chronic infections requiring long-term treatment or for those where preventative measures are unavailable or unaffordable.

Consider the case of malaria, a disease that disproportionately affects the poorest populations. The World Health Organization estimates billions of dollars are spent annually on malaria control, encompassing the costs of diagnostics, medications, and vector control initiatives. While these investments are crucial for disease control, the economic toll extends far beyond these direct expenses. The productivity losses from malaria, both in terms of workdays missed and decreased agricultural output, represent a significant impediment to economic development in endemic regions. The indirect costs associated with the long-term health consequences of malaria, such as neurological damage or chronic anemia, further amplify the economic burden.

Beyond malaria, other parasitic infections inflict substantial economic damage. Schistosomiasis, for instance, leads to significant morbidity and reduced productivity, particularly among children and working-age adults. The long-term effects of schistosomiasis, such as liver damage and bladder cancer, necessitate substantial healthcare expenditure. The economic consequences of soil-transmitted helminths, such as hookworms and roundworms, are also substantial, contributing to impaired cognitive development in children and diminished workforce participation in adults. These infections often affect populations in areas where poverty is already rampant, creating a vicious cycle of disease, poverty, and underdevelopment.

Investing in effective antiparasitic drug development and implementation is not merely a matter of public health; it's a sound economic strategy. The return on investment from preventing and treating parasitic diseases can be significant. Reduced healthcare costs, increased productivity, and improved human capital all contribute to substantial economic benefits. Strategies that promote access to affordable and effective treatments, coupled with improved sanitation and preventative measures, can yield significant economic returns in both the short and long term. Furthermore, the development of novel, cost-effective drugs and diagnostics is crucial to reduce the financial burden associated with parasitic disease management. This underscores the importance of collaboration between pharmaceutical companies, researchers, and governments to prioritize the development and equitable distribution of affordable antiparasitic medications.

The economic analysis of parasitic diseases should not only focus on direct costs but also account for the wider societal impacts. Loss of education due to illness, reduced agricultural output, and increased healthcare system strain are all crucial factors to consider when evaluating the total economic burden. The cost-effectiveness of various interventions, such as mass drug administration programs versus targeted interventions, should be carefully evaluated to optimize resource allocation and maximize economic impact. Developing comprehensive economic models that incorporate these various factors is critical for informed decision-making and efficient resource allocation in the fight against parasitic diseases. This requires a more holistic approach integrating economic analysis with epidemiological data and public health strategies. Only through a comprehensive economic evaluation of parasitic diseases can we effectively advocate for and implement sustainable solutions. This includes not only funding research and development of new treatments but also supporting infrastructure development and public health campaigns in affected regions.

In conclusion, the economic implications of parasitic diseases are multifaceted and far-reaching, posing a substantial challenge to global health and economic development. Addressing this challenge demands a multi-pronged approach that includes not only the development of novel and effective treatments, but also focuses on equitable access, sustainable control measures, and a nuanced understanding of the economic burden. This requires collaborative efforts between governments, international organizations, researchers, and pharmaceutical companies to address both the immediate health concerns and the long-term economic consequences of parasitic infections. Only through such a coordinated effort can we hope to meaningfully reduce the crippling economic impact of these diseases and contribute to a healthier and more prosperous world.

www.ingramcontent.com/pod-product-compliance
Lightning Source LLC
LaVergne TN
LVHW022012200926
848481LV00007B/2358